Extreme Careers™

Forensic Scientists

Life Investigating Sudden Death

Suzanne J. Murdico

rosen central™

The Rosen Publishing Group, Inc., New York

For my in-laws, Vince and Audrey Murdico

Published in 2004 by The Rosen Publishing Group, Inc.
29 East 21st Street, New York, NY 10010

First Edition

Library of Congress Cataloging-in-Publication Data

Murdico, Suzanne J.
Forensic scientists : life investigating sudden death / by Suzanne J. Murdico.— 1st ed.
p. cm. — (Extreme careers)
Summary: Examines the careers available in the field of forensics, discussing the necessary education, training, and on-the-job duties.
Includes bibliographical references and index.
ISBN 0-8239-3966-9 (libr. bdg. : alk. paper)
1. Forensic pathology—Vocational guidance—Juvenile literature.
[1. Forensic pathology—Vocational guidance. 2. Vocational guidance.] I. Title. II. Series.
RA1063.4 .M87 2003
616.07'023—dc21

2002153673

Manufactured in the United States of America

Contents

Introduction: Solving Mysteries 4
1 Searching for Clues 8
2 Analyzing Evidence 19
3 Cracking Cases 33
4 Forensic Specialties 42
Glossary 53
For More Information 55
For Further Reading 58
Bibliography 60
Index 62

Introduction: Solving Mysteries

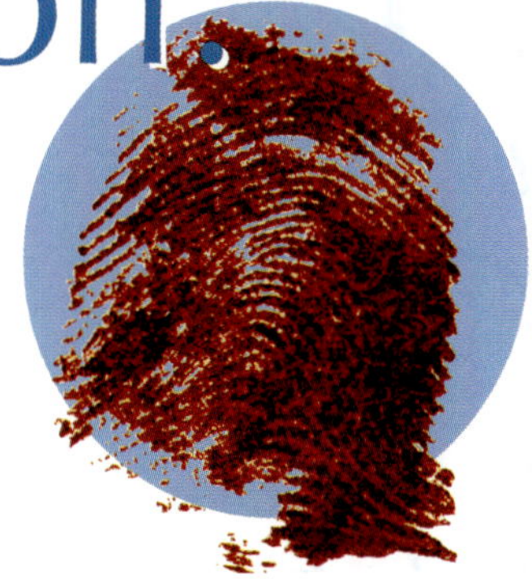

Richard Crafts thought that he had gotten away with murdering his wife, Helle. He even filed a missing persons report. He told police that his wife had left and not come back after an argument. Some of Helle's friends and relatives didn't believe Richard's story. They grew suspicious and asked the police to investigate.

The problem, though, was that Helle's body never turned up. How could investigators prove that Richard Crafts had killed his wife when there was no evidence that a murder had even taken place? Or was there?

Police soon got a break in the case. A snowplow driver remembered seeing someone who fit Richard Crafts's description running a wood chipper in the middle of the night. The police began to investigate further when they discovered that Crafts had in fact rented a wood chipper around the time of his wife's disappearance.

Investigators, including well-known forensic scientist Dr. Henry C. Lee, looked for evidence. They searched the area where the snowplow driver had seen the wood chipper being used. What the forensic scientists found was gruesome indeed—tiny chips of bone and teeth, and strands of blond hair.

Through forensic analysis, investigators determined that the evidence they found was the remains of Helle Crafts. Even though no body was ever found, Richard Crafts was convicted of murdering his wife.

The Role of Forensic Scientists

The word "forensic" comes from a Latin word meaning "public forum," or "court of law." Forensic science is the use of scientific knowledge applied to law. Forensic scientists collect and analyze evidence to help prosecutors prove in court whether a person did or did not commit a crime.

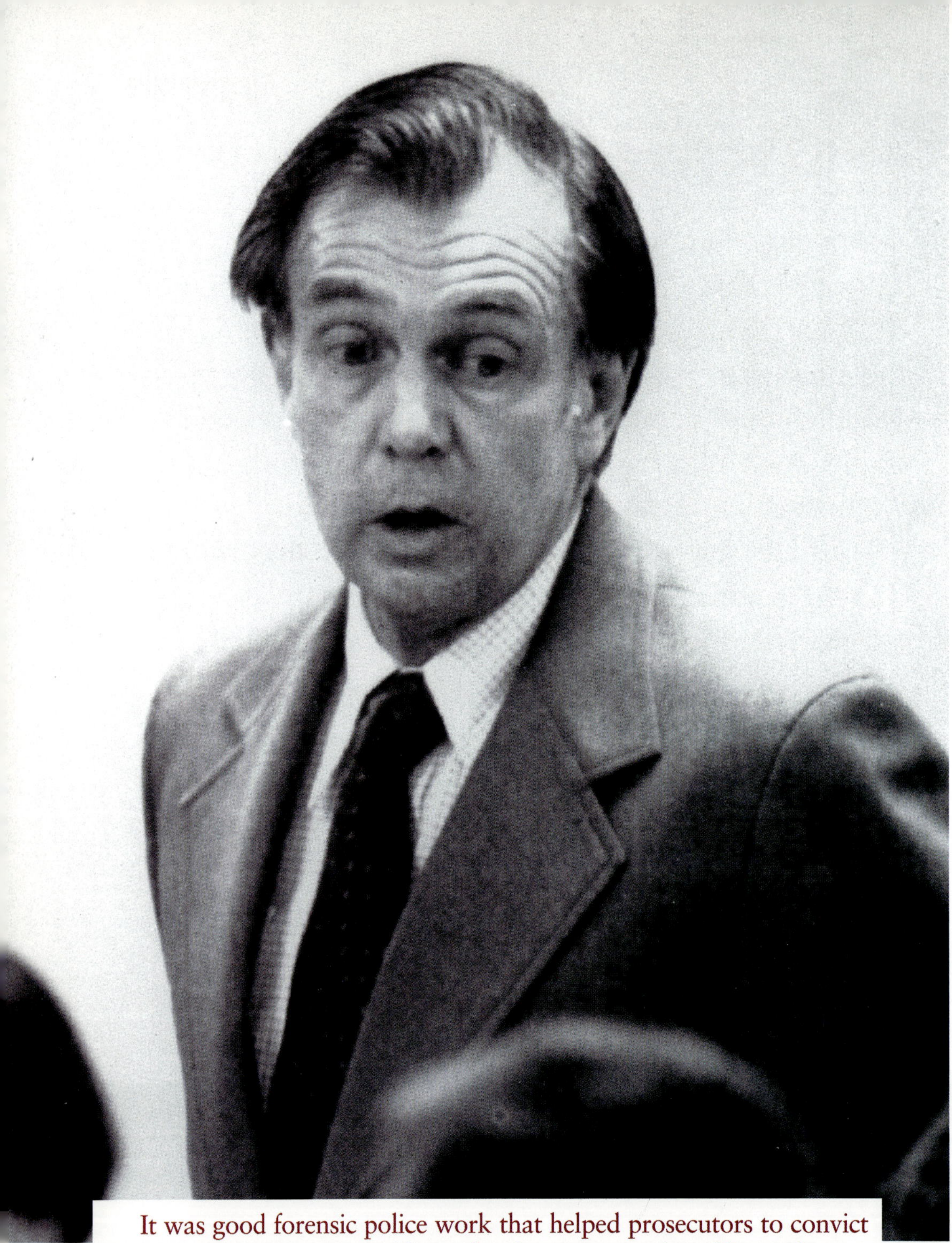

It was good forensic police work that helped prosecutors to convict Richard Crafts, pictured here, for the 1986 murder of his wife.

Introduction

Forensic scientists are probably best known for solving murders. Those are not the only types of cases they're asked to investigate, however. When any sudden or unexplained death occurs, forensic scientists are called upon to determine the who, where, when, why, and how of the case. In addition to murders, forensic scientists may investigate suicides and accidents, such as plane crashes or drownings.

Most of the work done by forensic scientists takes place in a laboratory. These experts play an essential role in criminal investigations. The goal of forensic scientists is to use scientific analysis to determine the facts and, as a result, the truth of each case. The work done by forensic scientists can help not only to put criminals behind bars but also to free people who are innocent.

Searching for Clues

1

One of the basic ideas of forensic science is that an exchange takes place during every crime. A person who commits a crime leaves something at the scene and, at the same time, takes something away.

The criminal may leave something nearly invisible, such as a fingerprint or a tiny bit of mud from the bottom of a shoe. No matter how small, though, it is evidence of the person's presence at the scene. By the same token, the criminal may unknowingly take away a drop of the victim's blood or a whisker from the victim's pet cat. Regardless of how carefully a criminal cleans the crime scene, clues remain for forensic scientists to find.

At the Scene of a Crime

Police officers are called to the scene when a sudden or unexplained death happens. First, the police look at the situation to decide if there is a threat to public safety. They must remove the threat if it exists. That could involve arresting a crime suspect if one is on the scene or making sure that the individual has already left.

Once the police have determined that the area is safe, the forensic scientists are called. At the scene, their job is to find all signs that might explain who committed the crime and how it happened. They search for clues to help identify the victim and the person behind the death. They also try to show a connection between the two. This evidence will later be used if the case is tried in a court of law.

It is necessary that forensic scientists use great care when searching for clues and collecting evidence. This care helps to prevent contamination and ensures that the laboratory analysis of the evidence will be accurate. It also proves the reliability of the evidence when it's presented in the courtroom.

Securing the Scene

You've probably seen crime scene tape on television news shows or in movies. It's yellow tape with the words "Crime Scene—Do Not Cross" stamped on it. This tape is used to mark the area where a crime was committed. Only authorized personnel, such as police officers and forensic scientists, are allowed past the tape.

Crime scene tape surrounds Pearl High School in Pearl, Mississippi, after a student killed two fellow students and wounded six others on October 1, 1997. The tape allows police and forensic scientists to work undisturbed.

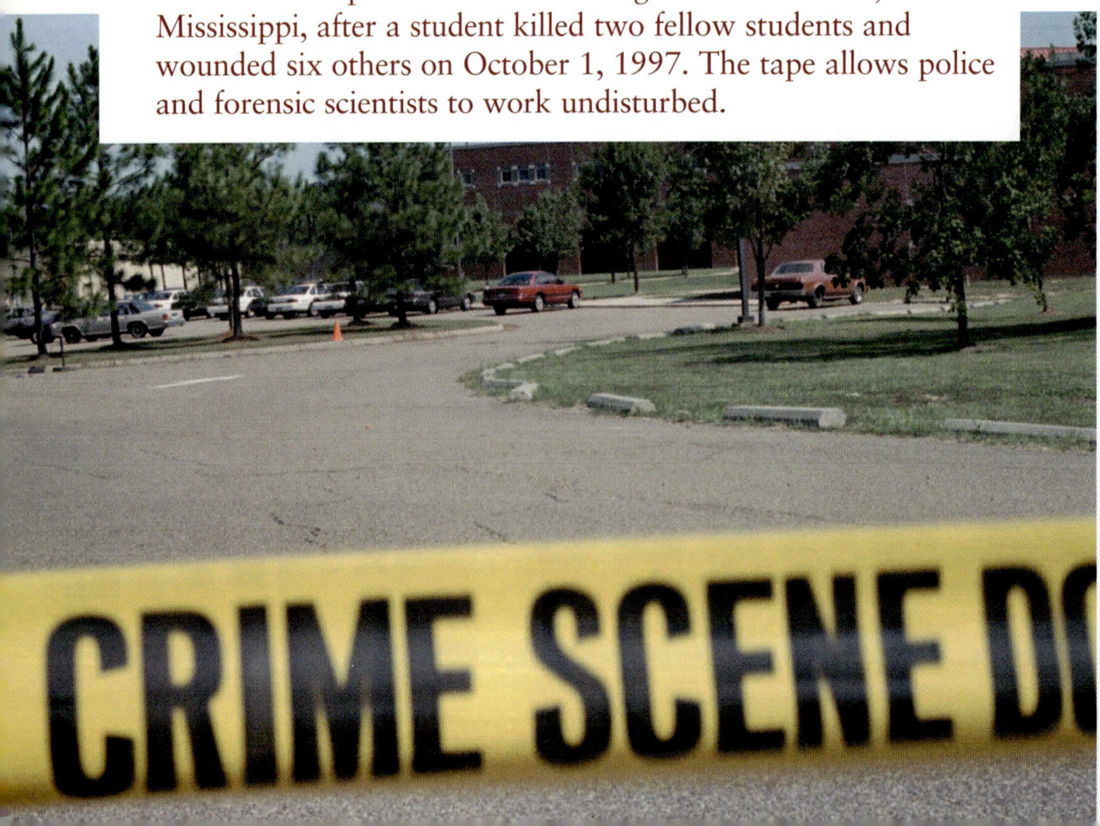

Using crime scene tape to secure the scene is the crucial first step in an investigation. Being able to "freeze" the crime scene allows investigators to find valuable evidence that could link a person to the crime. Curious neighbors, reporters, and other onlookers must be kept away from the crime scene so that valuable evidence is not accidentally lost or destroyed. If it is, a killer could go free.

Once the crime scene is secured, forensic scientists document it with photographs, videotape, and sketches. They also take notes about everything that they see—either written descriptions in a notebook or verbal descriptions spoken into a tape recorder. These notes contain just the facts, without analysis or opinions. After the crime scene has been carefully documented with everything in place, the collection of evidence can begin.

Collecting Evidence

The forensic team searches for any clues that might explain what happened and who is responsible. Clues

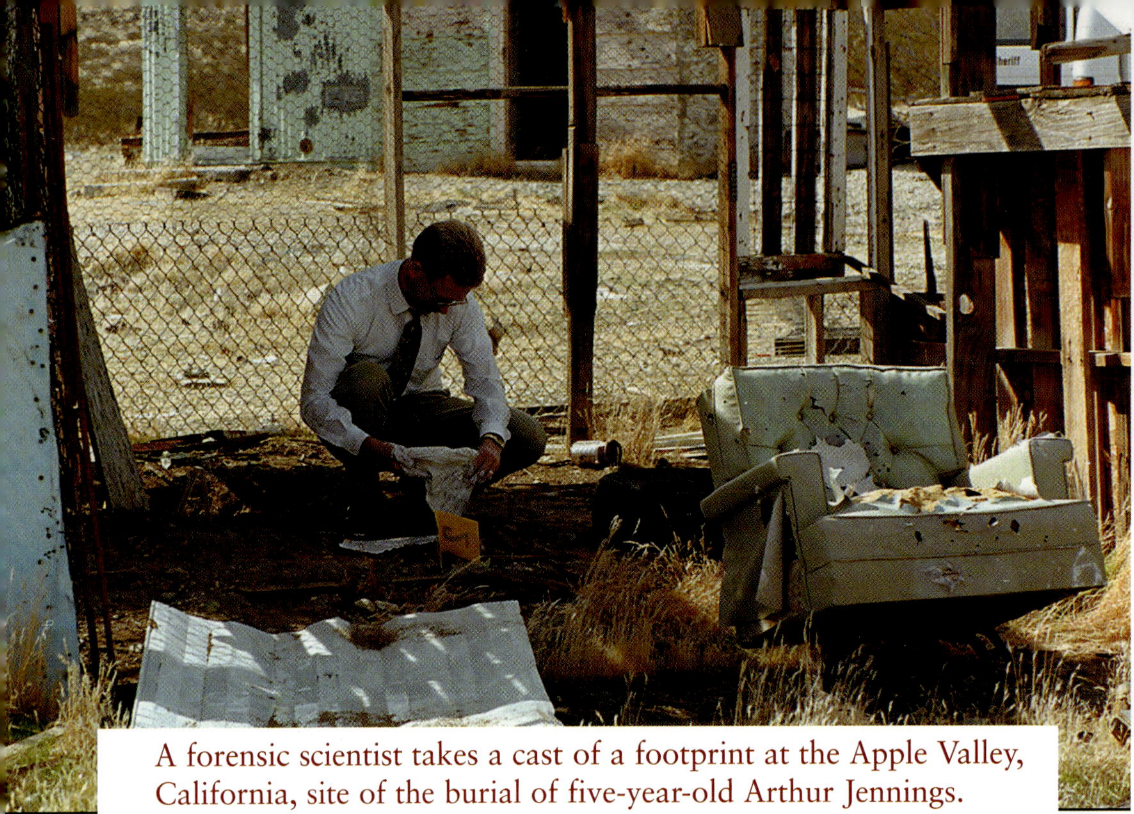

A forensic scientist takes a cast of a footprint at the Apple Valley, California, site of the burial of five-year-old Arthur Jennings. Jennings's parents were accused of his February 1996 murder.

might be as obvious as a smoking gun or a bloody knife. They could also be as subtle as a single strand of blond hair or a tiny blue carpet fiber.

Forensic scientists are responsible for collecting, processing, and analyzing these clues. At the crime scene, they gather every bit of evidence, being careful to retrieve even the smallest clue. Each item is packaged separately (to prevent one item from contaminating another), labeled, recorded, and properly preserved for future analysis.

Telltale Marks

A criminal sometimes leaves behind marks that only he or she could have made. These marks can help forensic scientists to accurately determine the person's identity. Fingerprints are one of the most common and most reliable types of telltale marks left at a crime scene. There are three types of fingerprints that might be found:

- Visible prints can be seen with the naked eye. They are usually left in a form such as blood, ink, or paint. Visible prints are also called patent prints.
- Plastic prints are impressions left in soft materials, such as clay or wax. They are also called molded prints.
- Latent prints are difficult, if not impossible, to see with the naked eye. They are created from oils and sweat on the hands.

To show latent prints, forensic scientists use a technique called dusting for prints. They spread a small amount of special powder across doorknobs, windows, light switches, or other surfaces that the criminal may have touched. The powder sticks to the fingerprint, and when the extra powder is brushed away, the fingerprint pattern can be seen. The forensic scientist then uses clear tape to lift the print from the surface. The print is placed on a print card for later identification.

In addition to fingerprints, other telltale marks might be found at a crime scene. For example, a criminal's shoes or car tires might leave tracks in mud or snow. A crowbar used to break into a home could leave tool marks on the window or door frame. Bite marks might be found on the skin of a victim or in food or chewing gum left at the crime scene.

In some cases, such as with bite marks in food, investigators can simply package the evidence and take it to the lab for analysis. In other cases, however, the evidence can't easily be moved. With tire tracks, for example, investigators first take a photograph of them. Then they make a plaster cast of the impressions and take the cast to the lab.

Bodily Fluids

Bodily fluids, such as blood, saliva, and semen, are often found at the scene of a crime, particularly a murder. Sometimes the bodily fluid is determined to

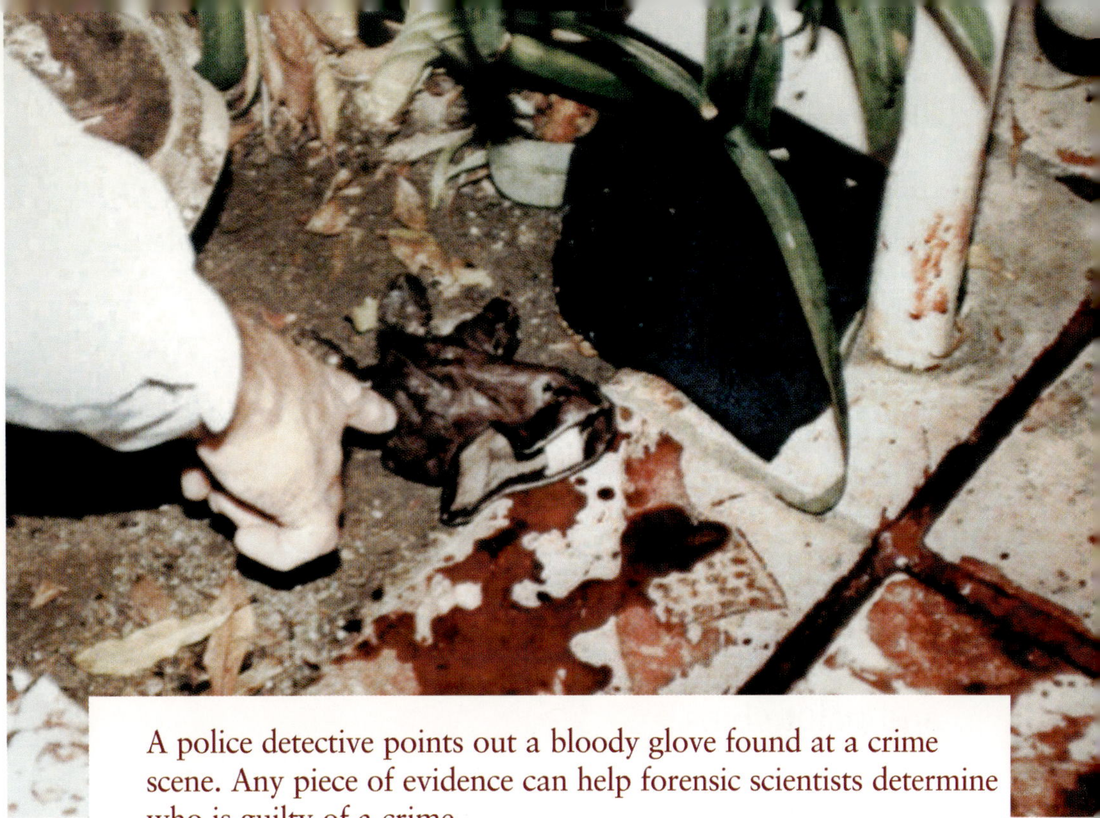

A police detective points out a bloody glove found at a crime scene. Any piece of evidence can help forensic scientists determine who is guilty of a crime.

belong to the victim, but not always. Sometimes it's a clue to the identity of the killer. For example, the victim may have scratched the attacker and gotten his or her blood under the fingernails.

Collecting blood and other bodily fluids can be tricky. Let's say that a bloodstain is found on a piece of clothing. If the blood is still wet, it should be collected in a paper bag and allowed to air-dry before it is analyzed. If the wet clothing were to be sealed in a plastic bag, the moisture could create mold or mildew. This would likely alter or even destroy the blood sample, making it unusable.

Tiny Clues

Besides obvious visible evidence, forensic scientists search for the tiniest of clues that might easily be overlooked. This type of evidence is known as trace evidence. Examples include strands of hair, clothing or carpet fibers, soil, gunshot residue, shards of glass, and paint chips.

The way in which trace evidence is collected depends on the substance. Hairs or fibers may be lifted with sterile tweezers or sucked up with a special vacuum cleaner. Dried soil or paint may be scraped off a surface using a special tool. Most trace evidence is stored in paper envelopes or bags.

Chain of Custody

One of the most important responsibilities of the forensic scientist is to maintain the chain of custody. This

Crime Scene Safety

There is no doubt that securing evidence and preserving the chain of custody are vital elements of crime scene investigation. Equally important, however, is the protection of the crime scene investigators against disease and injury.

The scene of a crime—particularly a murder—can be a dangerous place for forensic scientists. Some of the evidence they collect, such as blood, other bodily fluids, and used needles, may be infected with HIV, hepatitis, or other diseases. For this reason, it's essential for all crime scene investigators to take precautions to ensure their personal safety.

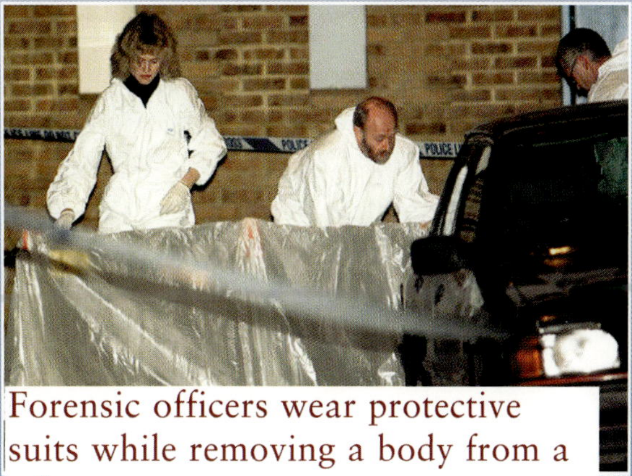

Forensic officers wear protective suits while removing a body from a crime scene.

These precautions include wearing protective clothing, such as latex gloves, foot coverings, coveralls, and goggles. In addition, investigators often wear respirator masks. These masks use special filters to prevent airborne particles, such as blood particles from scrapings, from entering the lungs.

chain is the process of documenting and protecting all evidence relating to a crime.

The chain of custody begins at the scene of the crime and ends in the courtroom, where the evidence is presented during a trial. At every point in between, the chain shows where the evidence is located and who has handled it. If the chain is ever broken or the evidence misplaced, the judge in the case may decide that the evidence has been spoiled. He or she may rule that it can't be used in court against the accused. More than once, open-and-shut criminal cases have been lost because of a break in the chain of custody.

Analyzing Evidence

2

Finding and gathering evidence at a crime scene is only the first step in the forensic scientist's attempt to solve a crime. The challenge really begins at the crime laboratory. There, the evidence found at the crime scene is examined, tested, and compared.

In the Crime Lab

The forensics work that takes place in a crime lab is called criminalistics. The scientists who work there are called criminalists. Many fields of science, including anthropology, biology, physics, and chemistry, are involved in criminalistics work. Large crime labs usually employ many forensic scientists who each focus on one area. Smaller labs usually employ only a few forensic scientists who have a basic knowledge of many areas.

In the crime lab, criminalists use scientific equipment to carefully analyze evidence. This equipment includes microscopes, computers, and highly specialized instruments called spectrographs and spectrometers. Criminalists may also use chemical treatments on some types of evidence.

Forensic scientists use high-tech machines to discover and analyze clues. Here, a machine uses filtered green xenon light to detect trace chemicals that make up a fingerprint.

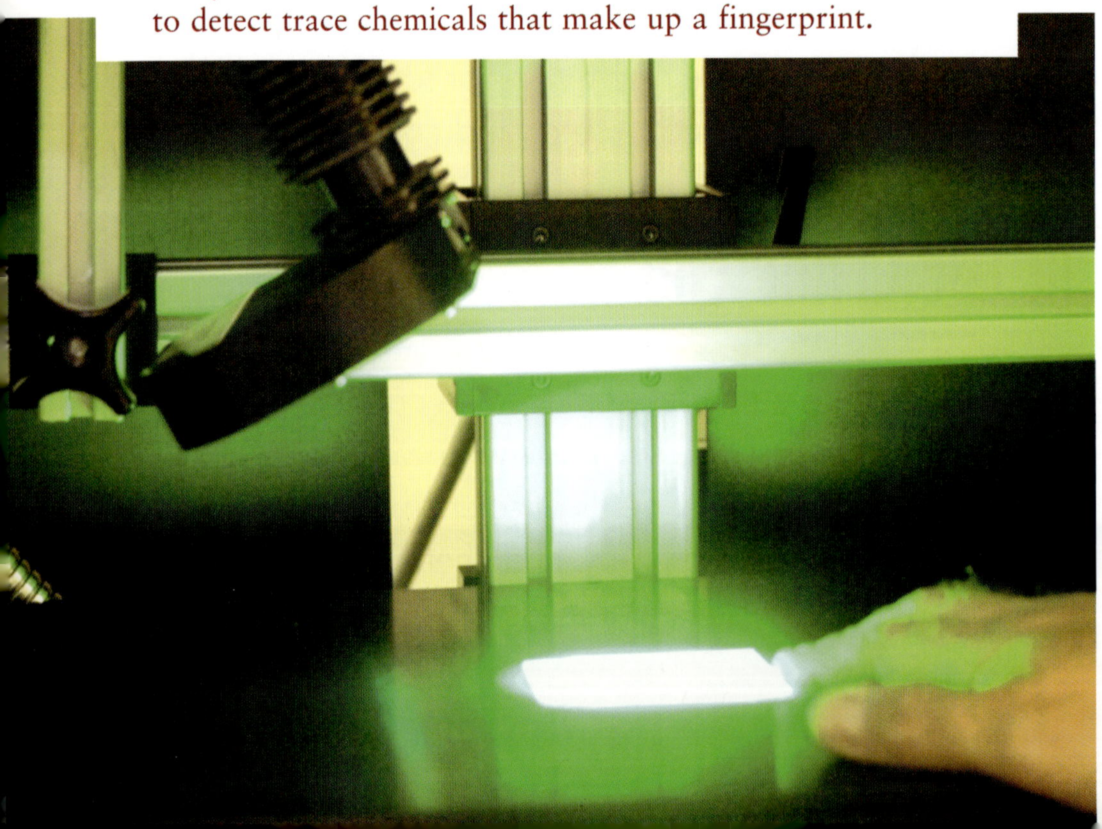

Physical Evidence

The characteristics of physical evidence can be divided into class and individual characteristics. Class characteristics are those that belong to a particular group of items. A certain brand of sneakers, for example, is a class characteristic. Individual characteristics are those specific to one particular item. The wear on the bottom of one person's sneaker is an individual characteristic.

Forensic analysis of physical evidence can determine both class and individual characteristics. A shoe print found at a crime scene, for example, might help investigators to estimate a suspect's gender, height, and weight. Specific characteristics, such as nicks or pebbles that appear in the shoe print, can be used like fingerprints and compared against a suspect's shoes.

Fingerprints

You may have heard that no two sets of fingerprints are exactly the same. Even identical twins have different fingerprints. With the exception of permanent scars, fingerprints remain the same throughout a person's lifetime. The fingerprints of a sixty-year-old man, for example, will look identical to those taken from the same man when he was fifteen years old.

Fingerprints have been and continue to be valuable clues for forensic scientists. They are one of the most reliable methods of identifying both the victims and the perpetrators of crimes. Although not always as reliable, shoe prints and bite marks can also be used for identification.

Before computers, fingerprint matching had to be done manually. Fingerprints left by a suspect were lifted from a crime scene and stored on a print card. Investigators then visually compared that set of fingerprints with millions of other identified fingerprints on file. If a match was found, investigators could place a specific person at the crime scene. As you might guess, sorting through millions of fingerprint cards was an extremely difficult and time-consuming task.

Today, fingerprints are scanned and stored on computers. Within seconds, the automated fingerprint identification system (AFIS) can compare a set of prints against millions stored in the nationwide database. The computer creates a list of prints that closely matches the original set. Then a fingerprint expert does a visual comparison to determine an exact match. The Federal

Print Patterns

Every person's fingers are covered with a pattern of ridges and valleys that creates a unique set of fingerprints. Although no two sets are the same, fingerprints can be grouped into four basic patterns:

1. Arch—a ridge that runs from one side of the finger to the other and has an upward curve.
2. Loop—similar to an arch but with a stronger curve; a loop turns backward and leaves the print on the same side it entered.
3. Whorl—an oval that spirals out from a central point.
4. Composite—a combination of the other patterns.

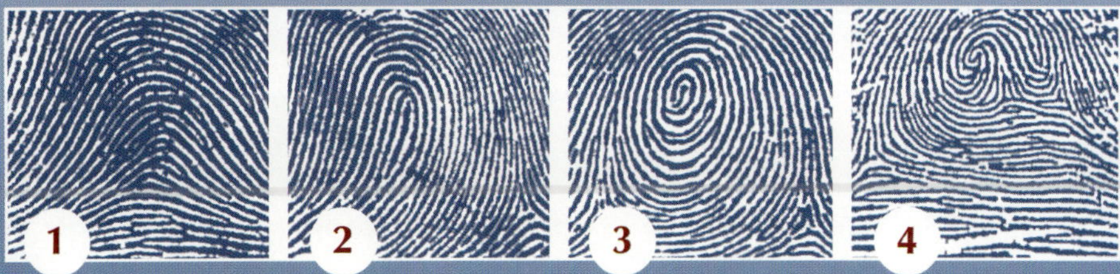

There are four basic types of fingerprints that include all the billions of prints present among people worldwide.

Bureau of Investigation (FBI) keeps more than 250 million sets of fingerprints on record.

Blood and Other Bodily Fluids

Years ago, blood could be matched only in terms of its type—type A, B, O, or AB. Over time, however, blood-testing methods improved. Specific elements in the blood could be detected, thus narrowing down the list of possible matches.

Today, blood testing is a highly sophisticated process. Much as fingerprints can, blood and other bodily fluids can now be used to positively identify

This forensic lab technician is testing bodily fluids to determine their genetic identity. Lab technicians wear protective gloves and uniforms so as not to contaminate the evidence.

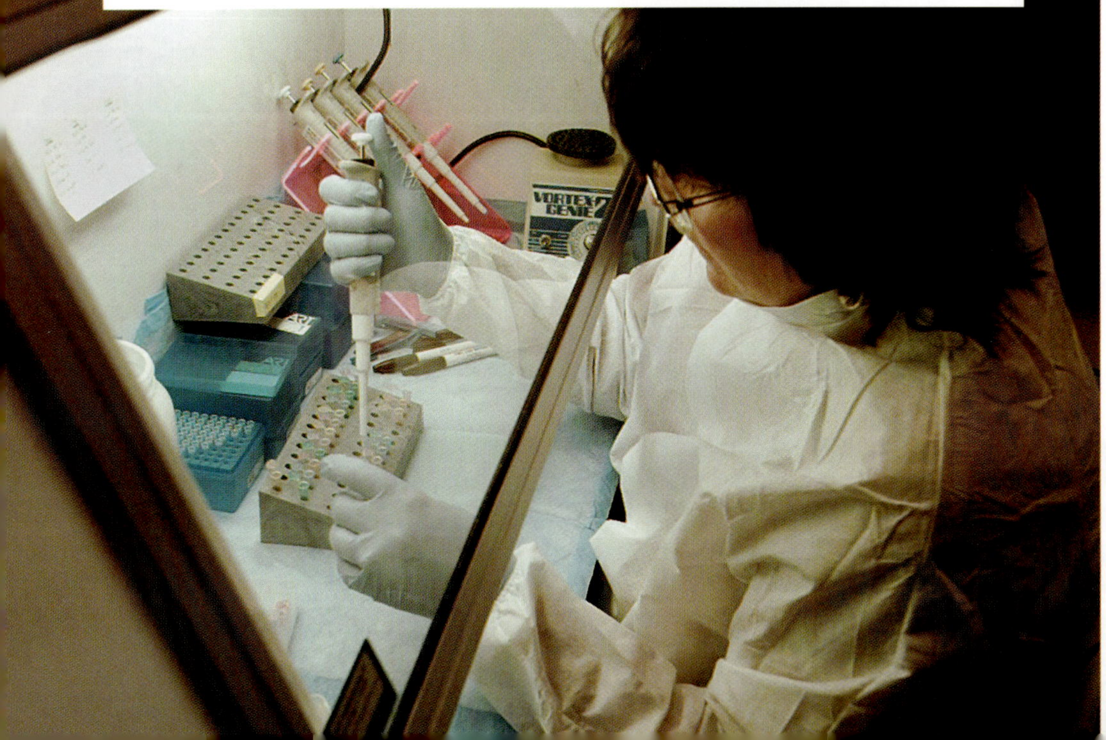

criminals. This is due to recent advancements in DNA technology.

DNA (deoxyribonucleic acid) is genetic material found in nearly every cell in the human body. Like fingerprints, each person's DNA is unique. DNA taken from blood or other bodily fluids collected at a crime scene can be compared with the DNA of the victim. If it doesn't match, the DNA can be compared with that of a suspect. This DNA analysis can either link a suspect to the crime scene or eliminate suspects.

Weapons and Tools

Criminals don't often leave murder weapons or tools at the scene of a crime. These items, however, are sometimes found later. They may be found dumped in a nearby trash can or stashed in the suspect's home. For a forensic scientist, a recovered weapon is a stroke of luck.

A bullet taken from a gunshot victim, for example, can be matched to the gun that fired it. In the same way, a knife can be tied to a murder even if the weapon has been carefully cleaned. With expert analysis, tiny drops of the victim's blood can still be taken from the knife. In much the same way, tool marks left at a crime scene can be matched to the tool used. If these weapons or tools can be traced back to a suspect, this will be solid evidence in court.

Trace Evidence

Tiny hairs or bits of fiber may be some of the most difficult types of evidence to locate at a crime scene. Under forensic analysis, this trace evidence can supply a surprising number of clues.

Hair

A single strand of hair can reveal a great deal of information about its owner. Analysis of a hair found at a crime scene can determine whether it came from an animal or a human. If the hair is from a human, forensic scientists compare it with the victim's hair. If it doesn't match, it could be a clue to the criminal's identity.

Forensic testing on a human hair can determine the person's race, the location of the hair on the body (head, chest, and so on), whether the hair was chemically treated (dyed or permed), and how the hair was removed (pulled, cut, and so on). It's even possible to determine whether the person used drugs or suffered from certain diseases. If the hair still has its root connected, further analysis can give more clues, such as the person's gender.

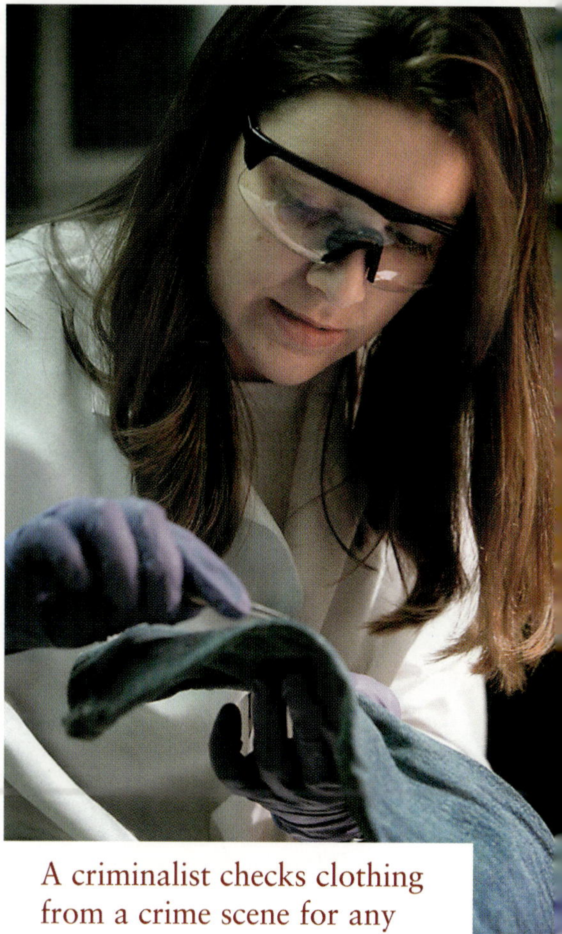

A criminalist checks clothing from a crime scene for any trace evidence of clues to help solve the crime.

Fibers and Other Traces

Analysis of fibers and other types of trace evidence can also uncover important information. For example, forensic scientists can determine whether fibers came from clothing, carpeting, or other materials. In some cases, they can even identify the manufacturer of the fiber. They can also compare it to fibers collected from a suspect's home or car to find a match.

Similar types of analysis can be done on soil samples, paint chips, glass fragments, and other minute particles. On its own, trace evidence may not be enough to convict a criminal, but it is often used to support other evidence during a trial.

Autopsy

One of the most important elements in a homicide investigation is the autopsy—an examination of the body after death. The autopsy often produces important clues that help to solve the case.

The autopsy is usually done by a medical examiner, a physician specializing in forensic pathology. The first step in an autopsy is to examine the outside of the body. Photographs and X rays are taken, and the body is weighed and measured. The medical examiner notes any injuries, such as bruises or knife wounds.

The Body Farm

More than a dozen dead bodies are strewn about the property. A chain-link fence topped with barbwire keeps out curious intruders. Exposed to the elements, the corpses are in different stages of decomposition. The stench of death is everywhere.

Although this may sound like a scene from a horror film, it's actually a real place. The Anthropological Research Facility at the University of Tennessee, Knoxville, is a one-of-a-kind laboratory. Known informally as the Body Farm, this facility provides the resources for forensic scientists to study corpses as they decompose. One of the most important goals is to find a way to more accurately determine time of death.

At the facility, the decomposition process is studied under a variety of conditions. For example, bodies may be left in the sun for hours, kept in the trunk of a car for days, or placed under water for a week or more. This research helps scientists to learn more about how to reconstruct the events surrounding an unexplained death. The corpses used for research at the Body Farm come from people who chose to have their bodies donated to science after their deaths.

He or she then collects any trace evidence, such as hairs, fibers, or bodily fluids, which may have been left by the killer.

Following the external examination, the medical examiner makes cuts into the dead body. These incisions give access to the internal organs. Each organ is examined and weighed, and the stomach and intestines are opened to reveal their contents. The medical examiner takes careful notes and sends any

Forensic scientists sometimes must cut into a victim's body to study the organs. Trace evidence of poison or drugs can be found in the lungs or liver. Internal bruises or bleeding can show the differences between natural death and murder.

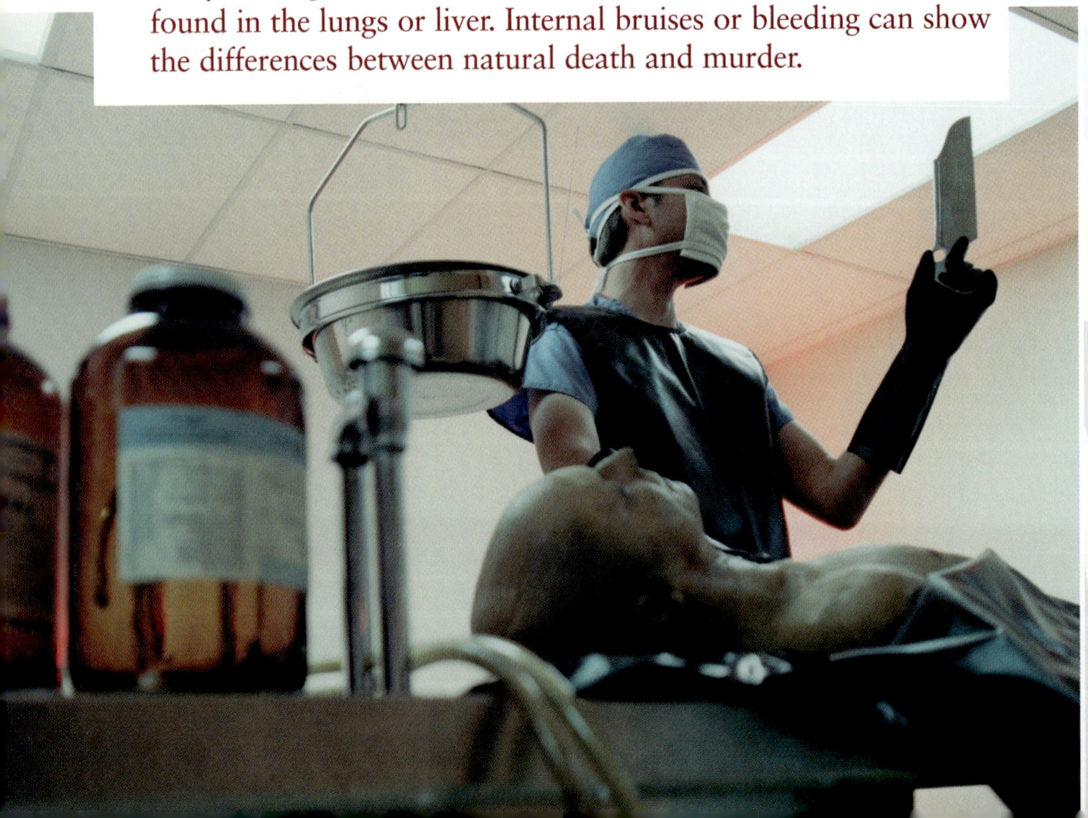

FORENSIC PROFILE: Dr. Michael Baden

For more than forty years, Dr. Michael Baden has worked in forensic pathology. Known and respected on an international level, Dr. Baden is one of the most prominent medical examiners in the United States. For many years, he worked in the Office of the Chief Medical Examiner in New York City. During his lengthy career, he has performed more than 20,000 autopsies.

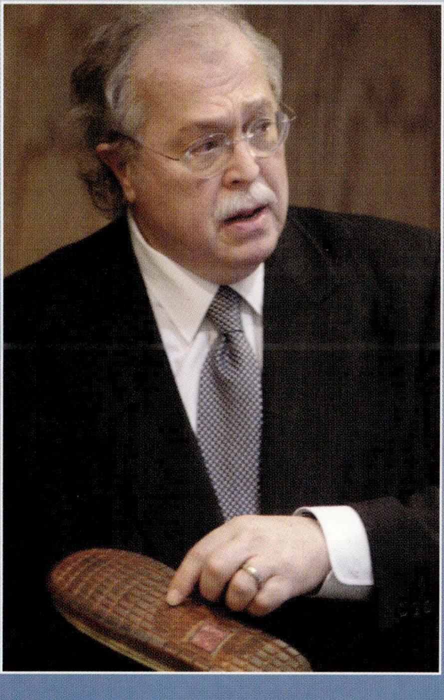

Dr. Baden has helped in the investigations of several high-profile cases. These include the homicides of Nicole Brown Simpson and JonBenet Ramsey. Dr. Baden has also acted as an expert witness in such cases as the death of actor/comedian John Belushi and the crash of TWA Flight 800.

In addition to his duties as a medical examiner, Dr. Baden has written two books about some of his most interesting cases. He also hosts the HBO television series *Autopsy*.

tissue or fluid samples to the lab for analysis. Then the organs are returned to the body.

From the autopsy results, the medical examiner determines the cause and manner of death. The cause of death is the physical condition that caused the death. The manner of death is the physical agent that led to the death. For example, the cause of death may have been massive internal bleeding, while the manner of death was a gunshot wound.

Cracking Cases

3

The ultimate goal of forensic scientists is to solve the mystery surrounding a sudden death. Cracking a case is like putting together the pieces of a puzzle. These pieces include the collection and analysis of physical evidence, the autopsy results, and the witness accounts.

To crack a case, forensic scientists must understand not only the rules of science but also the principles of logic. They need to create a theory about the crime and why it was committed based on the evidence. As new evidence is uncovered, the theory may change. But it should always show a logical cause-and-effect pattern that guides the investigation. In this way, forensic scientists work toward solving the crime and possibly identifying a killer.

Crime Scene Reconstruction

To solve a crime, it is important for forensic scientists to understand the sequence of events surrounding it. Based on the evidence they find,

A forensic team uses a mannequin to reconstruct the scene of the shooting of a teenager by police in Hartford, Connecticut, in 1999.

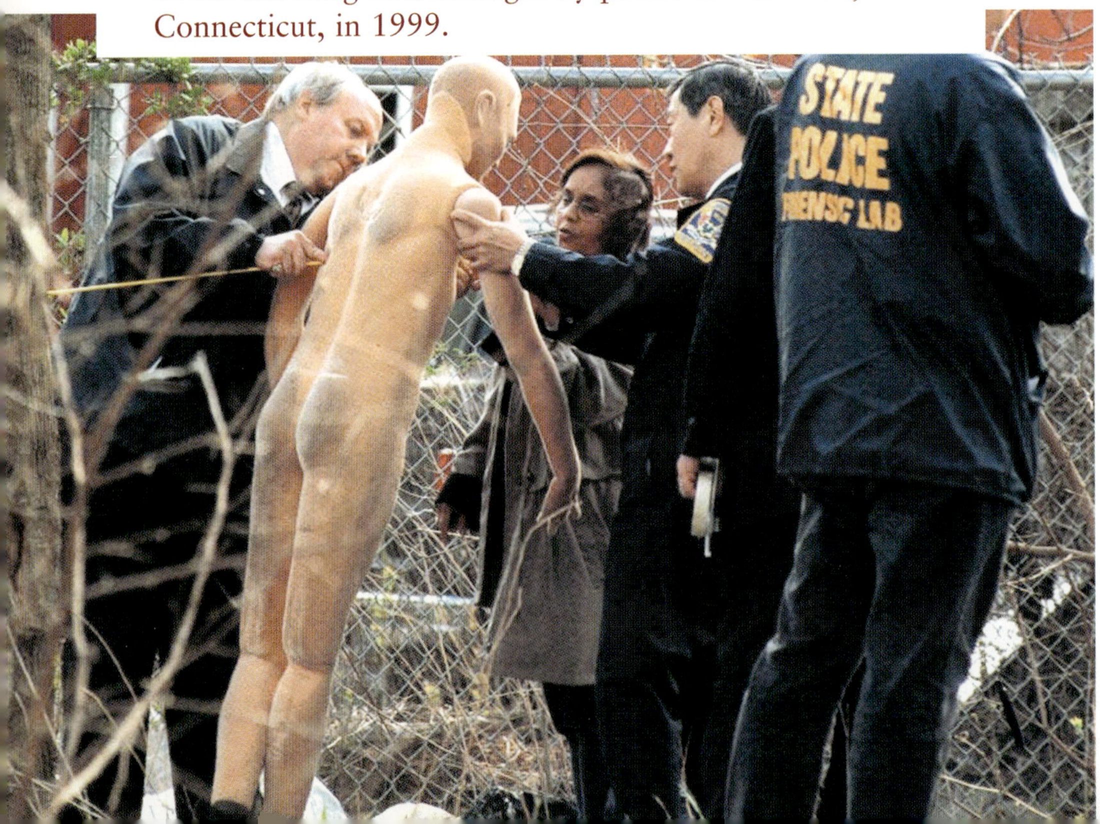

Criminal Profiling

The Boston Strangler. Son of Sam. Ted Bundy. Jeffrey Dahmer. The mere mention of these names strikes terror into the hearts of people everywhere. These men are examples of some of society's scariest criminals—serial killers. Serial killers often seek out people with something in common—for example, female nurses, college students, young men—and murder them for no apparent reason. The murders may continue for months or years.

The capture of some serial killers, including the Boston Strangler, has been aided by criminal profiling. Also known as behavioral profiling, criminal profiling is a technique used to dig into the psychological makeup of a criminal. In other words, profilers try to understand the killer's mind. They study a series of crime scenes and victims to figure out whether there's a good chance that the same person committed the crimes.

Experts in criminal profiling understand the signs and patterns of criminal behavior. They analyze the elements of a specific crime and combine them with this general knowledge. In this manner, criminal profilers can sometimes determine the characteristics of the killer. This information can help lead police to the person. In some cases, criminal profilers can even suggest ways for police to catch the killer.

investigators are often able to reconstruct the crime scene. This reconstruction can help them to develop a theory about the crime.

Suppose, for example, investigators determine that money and expensive jewelry are missing from a crime scene. They may suspect that the murder victim interrupted a robbery in progress. On the other hand, gunshot residue on a victim's hand and a suicide note may lead investigators to conclude that the victim took his or her own life.

Dan Roman, a police officer in Madison, Wisconsin, and an expert in bloodstain pattern analysis, stocks forensic equipment into the police department's crime scene vehicle.

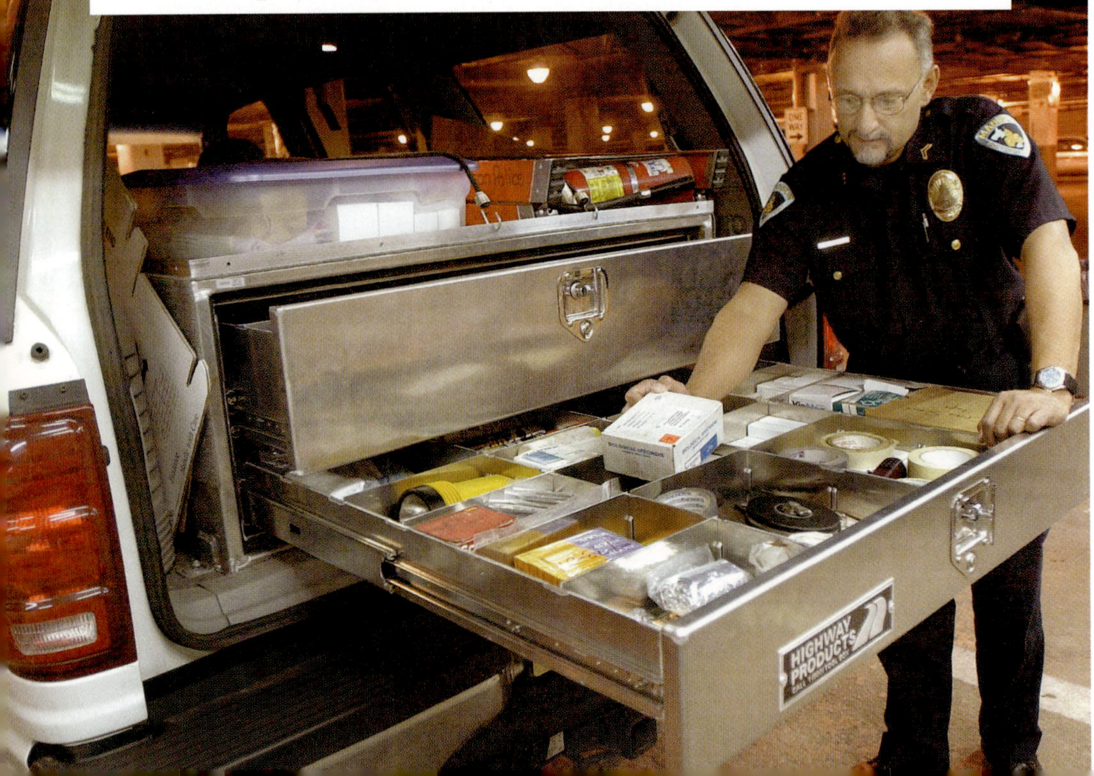

In some cases of violent crime, forensic scientists use blood spatter patterns found on the walls and floor to reconstruct the crime scene. They analyze the shapes of the blood droplets and the patterns of spatters to determine how the crime was committed. This analysis can provide many clues, such as the weapon used, the locations of the victim and the murderer, and the direction from which the attack came. Blood spatter patterns may even tell whether the murderer was right-handed or left-handed.

In the Courtroom

After all the evidence has been analyzed, forensic scientists usually have enough information to determine how and why a sudden death occurred. If a homicide was committed, they try to identify the person responsible. If investigators believe that they have enough evidence against the person, he or she will be arrested and charged with murder. Then the criminal trial begins.

Forensic Profile: Dr. Henry C. Lee

If you follow famous murder trials, you have probably heard of Dr. Henry C. Lee. Dr. Lee is a prominent forensic scientist who has been consulted for many high-profile cases. These include the murder trial of O. J. Simpson and the reinvestigation of the assassination of President John F. Kennedy.

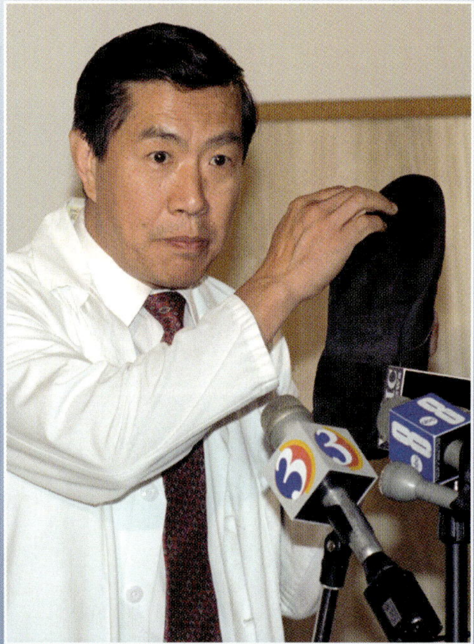

Dr. Lee was born in China and served as captain of the police force in Taiwan. In 1965, he moved to the United States to study forensic science. After receiving several advanced degrees, Dr. Lee worked at New York University Medical Center for nearly ten years. He went on to develop a program in forensic science at the University of New Haven in Connecticut.

Over the years, Dr. Lee has held several important positions. These include commissioner for the Department of Public Safety, chief criminalist, and director of the Connecticut State Police Forensic Science Laboratory. His work has taken him to thousands of crime scenes around the world.

Today, Dr. Lee serves as the chief emeritus for the Connecticut Division of Scientific Services. In addition, he teaches forensic science at the University of New Haven. There, he helped start the Henry C. Lee Institute of Forensic Science. Dr. Lee has also written many books.

Types of Evidence

During a trial, the prosecuting attorney tries to prove to the judge and jury that the person on trial committed the crime. Four types of evidence may be admitted in court:

- Direct evidence refers to the observations of an eyewitness to the crime.
- Physical evidence is any real object, such as a gun, shoe print, or clothing fiber.
- Circumstantial evidence is indirect information that may help to prove or disprove a theory.
- Testimony is a statement made by a witness, under oath, in a court of law.

DNA: Freeing the Innocent

DNA testing started in 1989, and it has revolutionized the criminal justice system. As important as it is for proving guilt, DNA testing is equally important for proving innocence.

Since the death penalty was reinstated in 1976, nearly 100 people on death row have been proven innocent. Of these 100, about 10 percent were freed through DNA testing. In some of these cases, DNA testing has also led to the identification of the real criminal.

Providing Testimony

Forensic scientists are often called upon to provide testimony during a criminal trial. The testimony made by an ordinary or fact witness is different from that of a forensic scientist. An ordinary witness can testify based only on what he or she saw or heard. An ordinary witness is not allowed to provide opinions about what happened. A forensic scientist, on the other hand, is considered an expert witness. He or she can be asked to provide testimony for either the prosecution or the defense.

Expert Witness

The testimony of an expert witness can include informed opinions based on evaluation of the evidence and interpretation of the scientific tests performed. An expert witness gives factual details about the evidence. He or she also explains the importance of the evidence.

A person must meet certain qualifications to be an expert witness. These requirements are based on educational degrees earned and length of job experience. They also include books or articles in professional journals that the person has written and membership in professional associations.

In the role of expert witness, the forensic scientist must be able to explain complex scientific ideas to anyone. On the witness stand, the forensic scientist will be speaking to a judge, jury, and lawyers who most likely don't have scientific backgrounds. The forensic scientist must be able to convert complicated scientific descriptions into simple terms.

As an expert witness, the forensic scientist must be fair and objective. He or she must tell the truth, whether it helps to convict or to free the defendant. All expert opinions must be based on solid scientific evidence.

Forensic Specialties 4

Forensic science is a large and diverse field. There is a variety of opportunities for those interested in pursuing a career in this exciting line of work. While some forensic scientists study bones or teeth, for example, others analyze blood or even bugs. No matter which specialty is chosen, however, the goal of all forensic scientists is the same—to unlock the mysteries surrounding a sudden death.

Forensic Pathology

While pathology is the study of disease, forensic pathology refers to the specific area of death and its causes.

All forensic pathologists are medical doctors. Forensic pathology is one of the most well-known fields of forensic science. One reason is that forensic pathologists are often portrayed in television crime dramas, since they are the specialists who do autopsies on crime victims.

The autopsy is one of the most important elements of a homicide investigation. Clues to a victim's identity, the cause of death, and even the identity of the killer are often revealed during an autopsy. It's the responsibility of the forensic pathologist not only to find these clues but also to analyze and interpret them for use during a criminal trial.

Forensic Anthropology

When it comes to skeletons, forensic anthropologists are the experts. Using human skeletons, they can help identify a person who died only a year earlier or one that died twenty years ago. Even a few bones can "speak" to a forensic anthropologist who knows how to listen.

Examination of a pelvic bone, for example, can establish whether the person was male or female. Studying bones in the legs and arms can reveal the

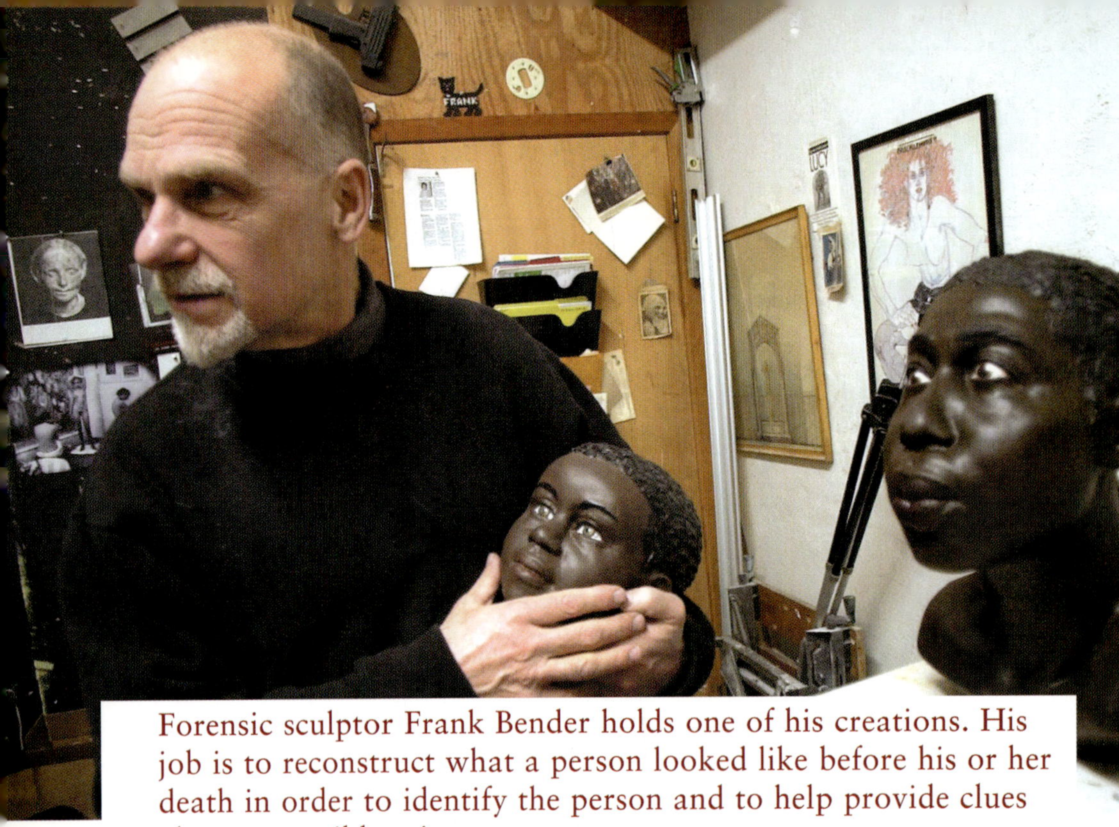

Forensic sculptor Frank Bender holds one of his creations. His job is to reconstruct what a person looked like before his or her death in order to identify the person and to help provide clues about a possible crime.

person's height and build. Bones in the hand indicate whether the person was right-handed or left-handed. Forensic anthropologists can also determine a person's age, race, and health status. In some cases, a person's bones even reveal clues about the cause of death.

Forensic Toxicology

Toxicology is the study of the harmful effects of drugs, chemicals, and poisons on the human body. Forensic toxicology, then, is the analysis of these findings for use in a criminal case. For example, a forensic toxicologist could determine if someone who died in a car crash had been driving while under the influence of drugs or alcohol. The skills of a forensic toxicologist might also be used to determine if someone was the victim of a drug overdose or a poisoning.

Forensic Odontology

Also called forensic dentistry, forensic odontology is the study of teeth to identify human remains. If a human skull is discovered, for example, it's impossible to identify the person based on a visual comparison. A forensic odontologist may be called upon to identify the person based on dental records. In this case, the forensic odontologist might search for a match by comparing the dental records from the skeleton against those of missing persons from the area.

In the event of a catastrophe, such as the crash of a jet airliner or the terrorist attacks on the World Trade Center, the work of forensic odontologists is vital. For the families of the victims of such tragedies, forensic odontologists bring a much-needed sense of closure by identifying their loved ones.

Forensic Entomology

If a person dies or is killed outdoors, insects will arrive at the scene within a few hours of death. It's the job of a forensic entomologist to study these insects, which include maggots, flies, and beetles. These tiny bugs can provide a surprising amount of evidence about a crime, such as the time and location of the victim's death. Sometimes a blood-sucking insect, such as a mosquito or chigger, can even help investigators identify the criminal by providing his or her DNA.

This information is not easy to determine, however. Many factors at a crime scene, including time of day, temperature, and exposure to sunlight or rain, will affect the insects living there. Forensic entomologists understand these factors and use them to determine the growth rate of the insects. From this growth rate, they can gather clues about the crime.

Fictional Forensics

Many people enjoy a good whodunit murder mystery. Dating back to the fictional detective Sherlock Holmes and mysteries written by Agatha Christie, people have always loved to read about crime solving. Some contemporary novels portray forensic scientists as the main characters. For example, a series of books written by Patricia Cornwell feature a fictional medical examiner named Dr. Kay Scarpetta.

Fictional forensics isn't limited only to books, however. In recent years, forensic science has become a popular subject on television. Dramas such as *CSI: Crime Scene Investigation* and *Crossing Jordan* showcase the work of fictional forensic scientists.

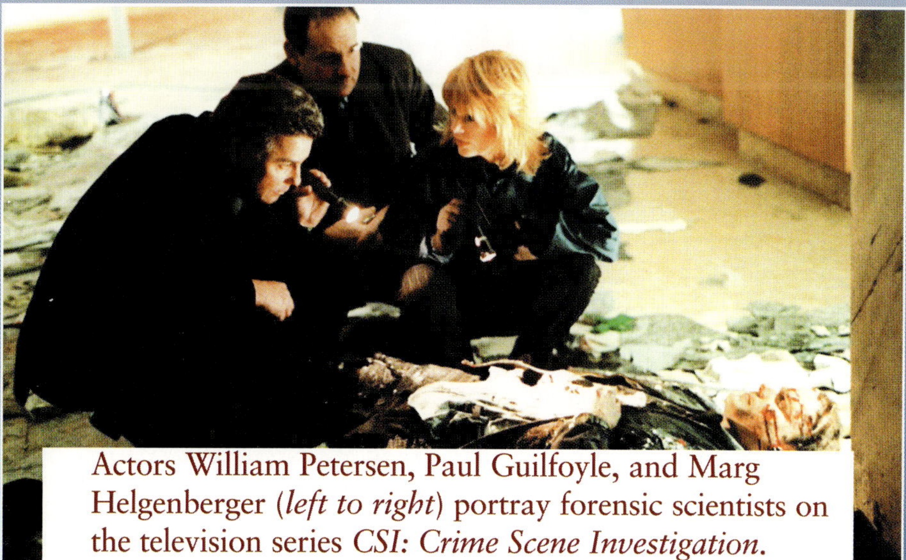

Actors William Petersen, Paul Guilfoyle, and Marg Helgenberger (*left to right*) portray forensic scientists on the television series *CSI: Crime Scene Investigation*.

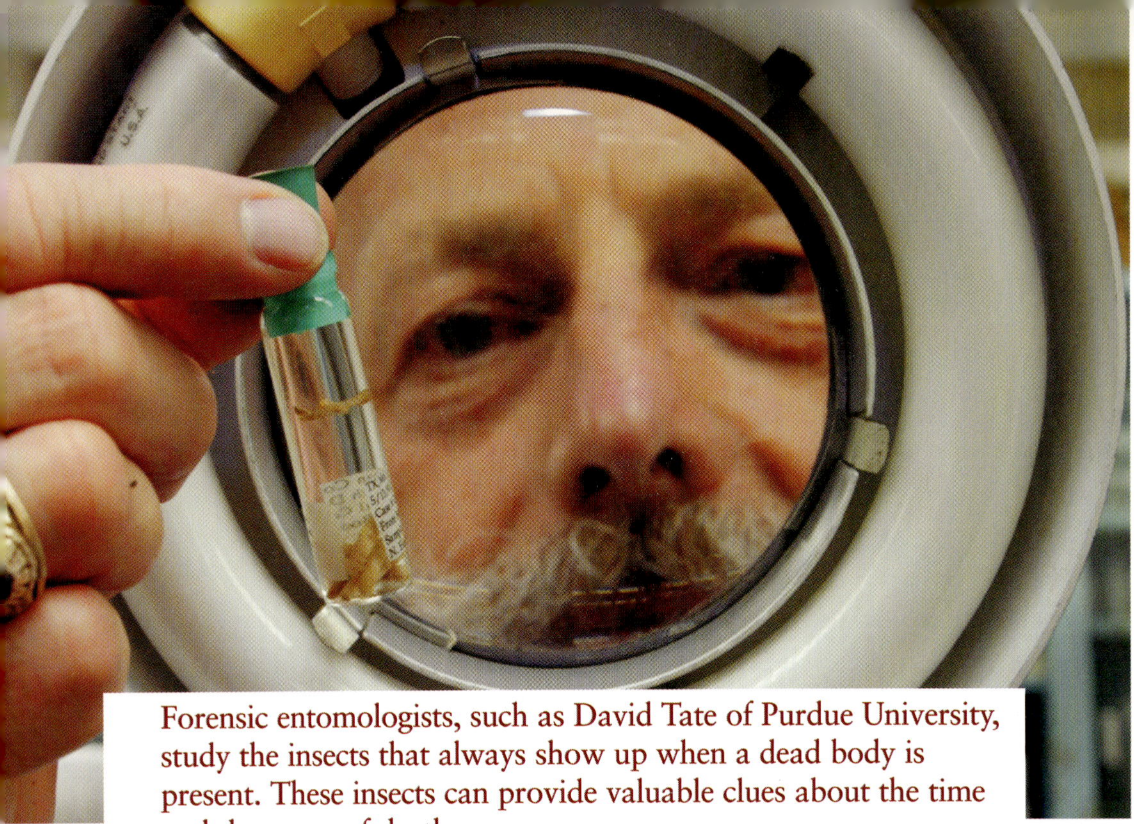

Forensic entomologists, such as David Tate of Purdue University, study the insects that always show up when a dead body is present. These insects can provide valuable clues about the time and the cause of death.

A Forensic Science Career

Some forensic scientists are employed by local government agencies, including police departments and county sheriff's offices. Others may work for state or federal government agencies. The FBI is one of the largest and most well-known employers of forensic scientists.

A career in forensic science is not for everyone, though. It's certainly not for the squeamish. Every day, forensic scientists stare down the face of death and confront the dark side of human nature. But forensic scientists play a vital role in the criminal justice system. With their help, crimes are solved and dangerous criminals are locked behind bars. A career in forensic science can be challenging and demanding. But for the right person, it's also highly rewarding.

Educational Requirements

The majority of jobs in forensic science require a college degree. For many forensic careers, a bachelor's degree in chemistry, biology, or a related science field is needed. For others, such as forensic pathologist, a medical degree is required.

After accepting a position, most forensic scientists receive on-the-job training. They may also take continuing education courses throughout their careers to learn the latest scientific techniques used in their field.

Skills Needed

Anyone who wants a career in the forensic science field needs to be detail oriented and must have sharp analytical and reasoning skills. Excellent speaking

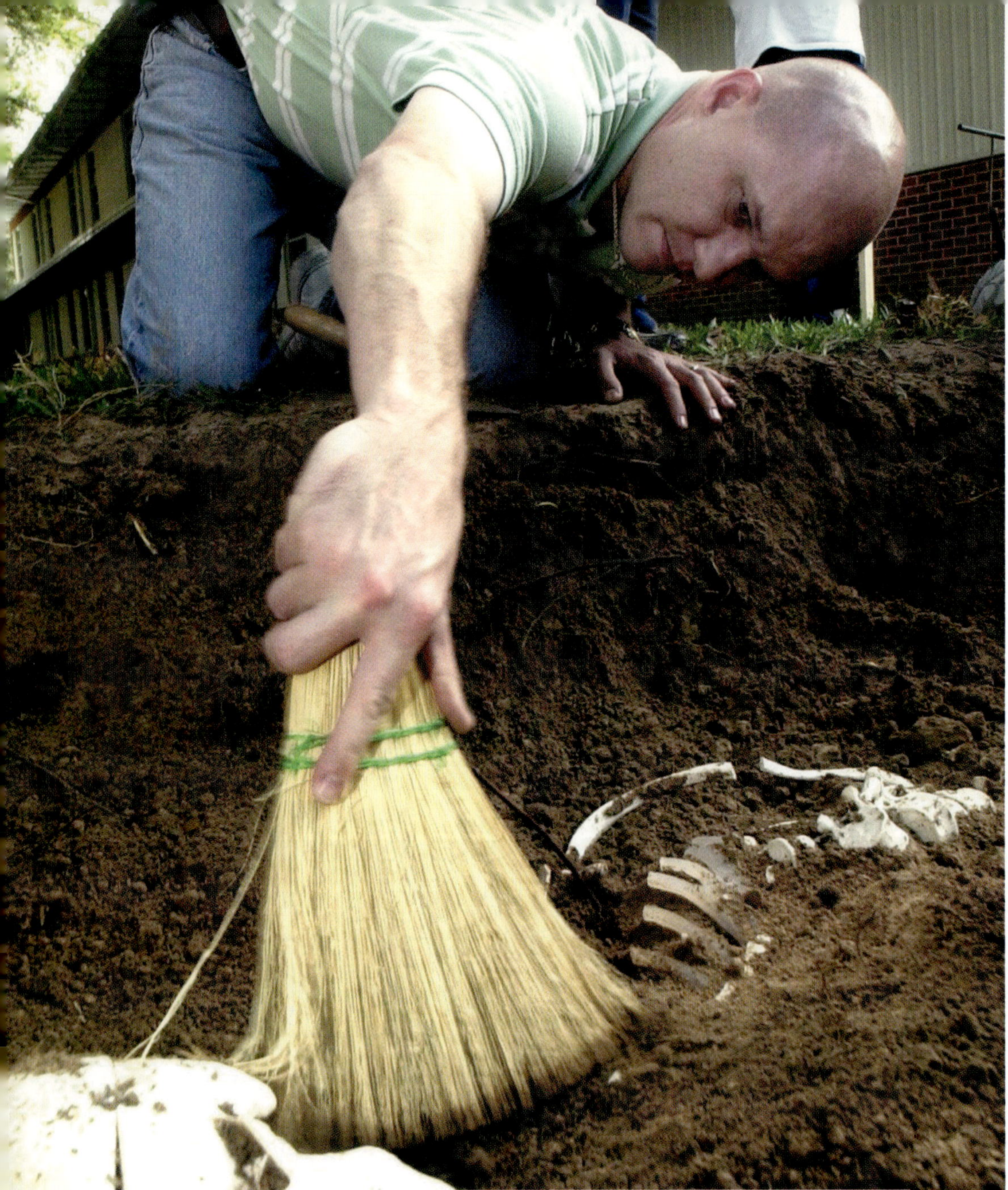

Forensic anthropology is the study of human bones that helps to determine time and cause of death. Here, Deputy Michael Sallow brushes dirt from a plastic skeleton during a class at the North Delta Police Training Academy in West Monroe, Louisiana.

and writing skills are also important for communicating information to colleagues, as well as to judges and juries in a court of law.

The job of a forensic scientist can be physically and emotionally demanding. Whenever a questionable death occurs—whether it's on a Sunday afternoon or at two o'clock in the morning—a forensic scientist may be called to the scene. The longer the evidence remains at a crime scene, the more likely valuable clues will be lost or destroyed. So forensic scientists must be available to investigate at a moment's notice.

Forensic scientists encounter death on a daily basis. The sight of violent crime scenes and accident or murder victims can be extremely disturbing. For these reasons, forensic scientists need the ability to be somewhat detached and to not become too emotionally involved in their work.

The Future of Forensic Science

As long as crimes continue to be committed, there will always be a need for forensic scientists to solve them. Advances in forensic technology, such as DNA analysis, have helped investigators to solve crimes and to catch criminals. But even these sophisticated techniques can't do the job on their own. They will never replace the role of the human forensic scientists who have the skills needed to interpret the information and present it in a court of law.

Glossary

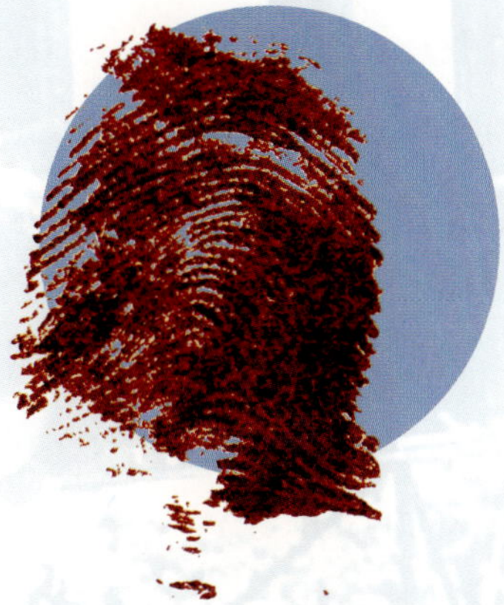

autopsy A medical examination of a body after death.

corpse A dead body.

criminalistics Forensics work done in a crime lab.

decomposition The process of decay or breaking down of a human being after death.

DNA Abbreviation for deoxyribonucleic acid; genetic material that is the basis for heredity.

evidence An object that gives proof of a crime.

forensic anthropology The study of skeletal remains that may have been involved in a crime.

forensic entomology The study of insects as part of a criminal investigation.

forensic pathology The medical study of human bodies that have been affected by crime.

forensic science The application of scientific knowledge to law.

forensic toxicology The study of drugs and poisons as they relate to a crime.

homicide The killing of one person by another person.

perpetrator A person who commits a crime.

suicide The taking of one's own life.

testimony A statement made by a witness under oath in a court of law.

For More Information

Organizations

American Academy of Forensic Sciences
P.O. Box 669
Colorado Springs, CO 80901-0669
(719) 636-1100
Web site: http://www.aafs.org

American Board of Criminalistics
P.O. Box 1123
Wausau, WI 54402-1123
(715) 845-3684
Web site: http://criminalistics.com/abc

American College of Forensic Examiners
2750 East Sunshine
Springfield, MO 65804
(417) 881-3818
Web site: http://www.acfe.com

Canadian Society of Forensic Science
2660 Southvale Crescent, Suite 215
Ottawa, ON K1B 4W5
Canada
(613) 738-0001
Web site: http://www.csfs.ca

National Association of Medical Examiners
1402 South Grand Boulevard
St. Louis, MO 63104
(314) 577-8298
Web site: http://www.thename.org

Web Sites

Due to the changing nature of Internet links, the Rosen Publishing Group, Inc., has developed an online list of Web sites related to the subjects of this book. This site is updated regularly. Please use this link to access the list:

http://www.rosenlinks.com/ec/fosc

For Further Reading

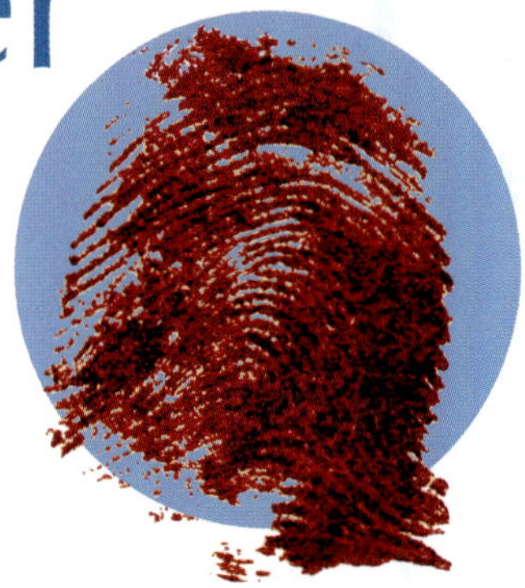

Bowers, Vivien. *Crime Science*. Toronto: Owl Books, 1997.

Camenson, Blythe. *Opportunities in Forensic Science Careers*. Chicago: VGM Career Books, 2001.

Campbell, Andrea. *Forensic Science: Evidence, Clues, and Investigation*. Philadelphia: Chelsea House Publishers, 2000.

Donkin, Andrew. *Crime Busters* (Dorling Kindersley Readers). New York: DK Publishing, Inc., 2001.

Friedlander Jr., Mark P., and Terry M. Phillips. *When Objects Talk: Solving a Crime with Science*. Minneapolis: Lerner Publications Company, 2001.

Jones, Charlotte Foltz. *Fingerprints and Talking Bones: How Real-Life Crimes Are Solved*. New York: Delacorte Press, 1997.

For Further Reading

Lane, Brian. *Crime & Detection* (Dorling Kindersley Eyewitness Books). New York: DK Publishing, Inc., 2000.

Woodford, Chris. *Criminal Investigation* (Science Fact Files). Austin, TX: Raintree Steck-Vaughn, 2001.

Yeatts, Tabatha. *Forensics: Solving the Crime.* Minneapolis: The Oliver Press, Inc., 2001.

Bibliography

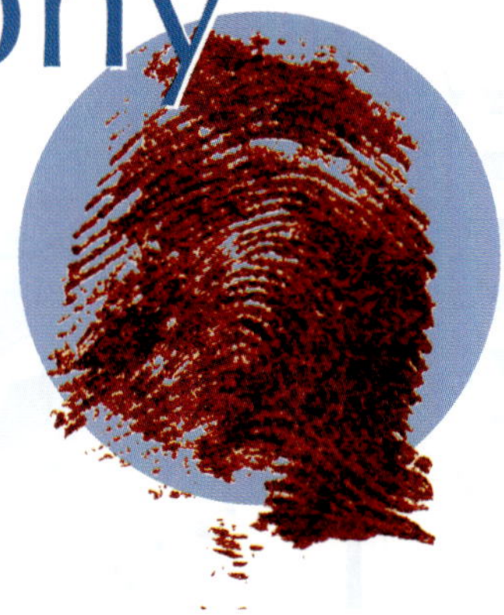

American Academy of Forensic Sciences. "AAFS Career Brochure." Retrieved June 25, 2002 (http://www.aafs.org/employ/brochure1.htm).

Campbell, Andrea. *Forensic Science: Evidence, Clues, and Investigation.* Philadelphia: Chelsea House Publishers, 2000.

Dillon, Hall. "Forensic Scientists: A Career in the Crime Lab." *Occupational Outlook Quarterly*, October 15, 1999.

Lundrigan, Nicole. "Crime Scene Priorities." *Law & Order*, May 1, 2001, page 38.

National Association of Medical Examiners. "So You Want to Be a Medical Detective?" Retrieved June 20, 2002 (http://www.thename.org/medical_detective.htm).

Ramsland, Katherine. The Crime Library. "All About Crime Scene Analysis." Retrieved August 2, 2002 (http://www.crimelibrary.com/forensics/crime).

Ramsland, Katherine. The Crime Library. "Crime Investigation Through Autopsy: Dr. Michael Baden." Retrieved August 2, 2002 (http://www.crimelibrary.com/forensics2/autopsy).

Ramsland, Katherine. The Crime Library. "Henry C. Lee Interview." Retrieved August 2, 2002 (http://www.crimelibrary.com/forensics/henry_lee/index.htm).

Rowh, Mark. "Hot Jobs in the Crime Lab." *Career World*, February 1, 2000, page 29.

Schiro, George. Crime Scene Investigation. "Collection and Preservation of Evidence." Retrieved July 30, 2002 (http://www.crime-scene-investigator.net/evidenc3.html).

Service, Robert F. "Body Chemistry: Where Dead Men Really Do Tell Tales." *Science*, August 11, 2000.

Thornton, John I. "Crime Laboratory." *World Book Encyclopedia* (2002), January 1, 2002.

Index

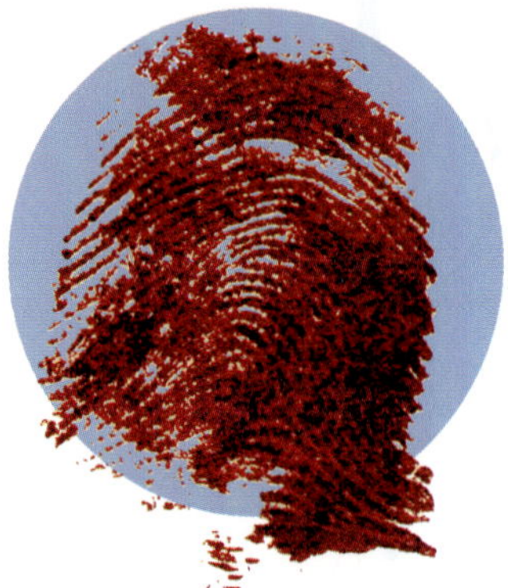

A

autopsy, 28–32, 33, 43

B

Baden, Dr. Michael, 31
blood testing, 24
bodily fluids, 14–16, 17, 24–25, 30
Body Farm, the (Anthropological Research Facility), 29

C

chain of custody, 16–18
crime lab, 19–20
crime scene
- documenting, 11
- reconstruction of, 34–37
- and safety, 17
- securing, 10–11

criminalistics, 19
criminal profiling, 35
criminal trial, 37–41
- evidence in, 39

D

DNA testing, 25, 41, 46, 51–52

E

evidence
- analyzing, 19–28, 37, 43
- collecting, 11–12
- finding, 8–16, 18
- left behind by criminals, 8, 13–16
- physical, 21–25, 33, 39
- telltale marks, 13–14
- trace, 16, 26–28
- types of, 39

F

Federal Bureau of Investigation (FBI), 23, 48

fingerprints, 8, 13–14, 21–23, 24, 25
dusting for, 13–14
forensic anthropology, 43–44
forensic entomology, 46
forensic odontology, 45–46
forensic pathology, 42–43
forensic science
career in, 48–51
definition of, 5
and fiction, 47
future of, 51–52
specialties of, 42–46
forensic scientist,
and cracking a case, 33–37, 49
duties of, 5–7, 9, 12
education for, 49
and safety, 17
skills needed, 49–50
forensic toxicology, 44–45

L

Lee, Dr. Henry C., 5, 38–39

M

murder, 4–5, 7, 14–15, 17, 25, 36, 37, 43

S

serial killers, 35
suicide, 7, 36–37

T

testimony, providing, 39, 40

W

weapons/tools, 25–26, 37
witness, expert, 40–41

About the Author

Suzanne J. Murdico is a freelance writer who has authored numerous books for children and teens. She lives in Florida with her husband, Vinnie, and their cat, Zuzu.

Photo Credits

Cover, pp. 6, 10, 12, 15, 17, 20, 24, 28, 31, 34, 36, 38, 44, 48, 50, © AP/Wide World Photos; p. 30 © Shuji Kobayashi/Getty Images, Inc; p. 47 © Everrett Collection.

Designer: Les Kanturek; Editor: Mark Beyer; Layout: Thomas Forget